To Bekai

M000114713

POETIC EXPRESSIONS IN NURSING:

Sharing the Caring

2nd Edition

SUSAN J. FARESE, MSN, RN

Yours in Nursing + Poetry!
Susan J. Farese
MSN, RN

ISBN: 978-1-7369776-1-3

Printed in the United States of America

Cover by: Lisa Shea

Published by: SJF Communications

Author photo by: Emmy Farese

DEDICATION

Dedicated to:

Nurses, and those who care about them…everywhere

and to my family and friends, past, present, future

"When it's all said and done, there's no profession as diverse,
as the art and the science of being a NURSE!"

-Susan J. Farese, MSN, RN

Table of Contents

AUTHOR'S NOTES 2021 and 1993

Poetic Expressions in Nursing: Sharing the Caring (2nd Edition)

AUTHOR'S NOTE 2021

Welcome to my 2nd edition of *Poetic Expressions in Nursing: Sharing the Caring* (2021) which was originally published in 1993. It's hard to believe that I began writing poetry in 1991, thirty years ago! More of my poetry writing and sharing journey is discussed in my note from 1993 which follows in the next section.

I have been licensed as a registered nurse since 1978. I received my Master of Science Degree in Nursing in 1986. Most recently (and after several reinventions), I am a communications professional but still utilize the nursing process with clients: assessment, planning, implementation and evaluation.

As one of the pioneers of nursing poetry, and after scouring the literature and networking with other nurse poets during the 1990s, I incorporated valuing the benefits of poetry as an informative, motivating, inspiring, stress management tool.

After *Poetic Expressions: Sharing the Caring* was published in 1993, I began teaching continuing education workshops for nurses to spread the awareness of how therapeutic and cathartic writing, sharing, and reading poetry can be.

This led me to teaching poetry as creative art to nurses throughout several states (1993-1997) as well as in Sweden (1994) and as a Distinguished Lecturer for Sigma Theta Tau the National Nursing Honor Society (1997).

Presently I teach Haiku workshops for the general public and since the pandemic have been teaching virtually.

My Author's Note from 1993 follows and it still rings true.

Yours in Poetry,

Susan J. Farese, MSN, RN

Poetic Expressions in Nursing: Sharing the Caring (1ˢᵗ Edition)

Each day, nurses experience an array of unique challenges, stressors, and ethical dilemmas as health care providers. Whether in a clinical environment, administrative, teaching, or non-traditional role, the nurse carries feelings deep within which may range from ecstatic highs to devastating lows.

Poetry, one of many creative arts, can be an enriching and therapeutic outlet for nurses in our personal and professional lives. Through poetry, our nursing experiences, thoughts, values, and feelings are explored, processed, written, communicated, and verified. Our insight and compassion regarding human behavior, health, illness, suffering, and death sharpens.

Through the avenue of poetry, nurses can uniquely *share their caring* and relate to others from all walks of life. Poetry in patient care, as well, can enhance the nurse's, client's and/or caregiver's psychosocial and spiritual well-being.

Nursing poetry can contribute to stress management, values clarification, strengthening the impact and image of nursing as a profession, and has extraordinary implications for further nursing research. Poetry, then, is an excellent tool for personal and professional development.

I welcome you to join me on the journey I've taken with nursing poetry. It has been cathartic, eye-opening, and enriching and actually happened by accident in March 1991, when I saw the movie *Awakenings*. One of the female characters (who caught the ball from her wheelchair) vividly resembled my maternal grandmother, Ann, who was an unfortunate victim of Alzheimer's Disease. She died, institutionalized, at age 60 in 1971, a time when support groups and resources were nil regarding this devastating illness.

Ann was very dear and special to me during my early childhood. Then from age 8-14, I witnessed the profound grief of gradually losing someone significant, with so much spirit and zest, before my eyes, before her time. It was confusing and frightening to see her regress to a vegetative, mute state. I know I was called to the nursing profession because of this early loss experience.

I repressed many of the deeply rooted feelings about Ann for nearly twenty years, until 1991, the night I saw *Awakenings*. Suddenly, that week, a three-page poem *Ann's Zest Ends* evolved which cascaded *from the heart*.

When I called my mother and read the poem to her, she as well shared many tears of relief, and asked, me to share *Ann's Zest Ends* with as many people as possible, because it so closely reflected what our family experienced with Ann's gradual loss. That was all I needed!

I began my crusade and presented the poem to several Alzheimer's support groups, nursing organizations and other community and professional groups. Ann's spirit and zest returned each time. Tears and tissue boxes appeared out of nowhere. I knew then that this message *connected* with so many people and related to them in their own way. The response was overwhelmingly positive.

This tremendous response gave me the confidence to continue writing poetry. In addition, I have provided many seminars and continuing education classes for nurses as well as the general public regarding poetry. This book is the culmination of my efforts.

I sincerely hope that you, the reader, not only enjoy "Poetic Expressions" but also pick up your pens and join me in the journey of self-discovery.

Yours in Poetry,

Susan J. Farese, MSN, RN

CONNECTION ON A BRIDGE

(To my patient)

Do you know, and realize and care?

That I, your nurse, know, realize and care…

about you, your personal condition, your beliefs
(of health's *ease* or *disease?*)

on you
your *loved ones* or your lifestyle?

Please ponder that, the next time you see me,
Scurrying about, from room to room,
Down one hall, or another
Passing medications, providing nursing care
and treatments
and using my *intuition*

In this,
The big, *little city* of the hospital
See that I know, realize, and care.
Allow me to enter, cross and reflect
On the bridge
That separates your world from mine
Share your world with me...
Don't be afraid…
Connect

NURSING IS

A: A chance to influence and inspire others; A chance to grow personally and professionally; the Art of Nursing

B: Being there when they need us (patients, peers, employers) – But knowing when to let go...

C: Caring, Choosing, Commitment

D: Deliberate attempts to make a difference

E: Eager and energized in our ethical actions

F: Facilitating others toward their paths of well being

G: Guiding others and ourselves towards goals and self-actualization

H: Harmonious peer relationships

I: Intelligence, Intuition, Inquiry, and Image

J: Joining forces with clients

K: Kindred spirits

L: Learning continuously to advance our skills, knowledge, and abilities

M: Meaningful interactions with clients; Mentoring those who need our expertise and wisdom

N: Not always needing to be in control! Never compromising our ethics, principles, integrity

O: Our reason for being nurses, our vocation

P: Professional as well as personable demeanor, Having a "purpose"

Q: Query if we're unsettled or if our intuition is uneasy

R: Respect for client and human rights; Risk taking

S: Sincerity, selflessness, self-confidence, self-esteem

T: Thorough, trusting, trustworthy

U: Universal precautions!! Unity in our image

V: Values that enrich ourselves and others

W: Worthiness when nursing is from the heart

X: eXperiencing diversity in practice

Y: Yielding sometimes but not always

Z: Zenith, Zest.

GIVING THANKS

Nurses know...

...the paleness and coolness of shock
...the dusky blue hues of cyanosis
...the significance of impending doom
...the fear in their eyes when fate is unknown
...the wails of terminal pain
...the scent of pseudomonas
...the tenacity of suctioned secretions
...the fruity breath of ketoacidosis
...the predictable patterns of Kussmaul breathing
...the jello-like non-rhythmic quality of ventricular fibrillation
...the bedlam in a code
...the frustration when a patient's noncompliant
...the intensity of patient care
...the thank yous that mean so much

BE THANKFUL, NURSES KNOW...

THE NURSE

If and when you thirst for comfort,
when your pain just won't subside,
Or your tears reveal the grief that you've been carrying inside...

Who's the person, calming all –
answering bells that beckon, call?
It's the nurse...there's no doubt, it's the nurse...

If and when you're one day post-op
And it's time to take a glance
At your fresh brand-new incision, body image un-enhanced

Who's the person near your side
With compassion one can't hide?
It's the nurse, there's no doubt, it's the nurse...

No matter when you have the need
Through illness, wellness, birth, or life's end
The nurse is so supportive, simply one of a kind
Whose comfort and knowing can mend

If and when you're in need for the quality of life
While all others may seem out of place
Call the nurse, heed the nurturing, caring, support
Blessed with wisdom, connection, and grace...

ANN'S ZEST ENDS

PRELUDE
Her zest for life, boundless energy
A smile a minute, so full of glee...
Remembrances of my grandmother Ann,
so significant to me.

She ran the show, she was "in the know"
About this or that, nonetheless, always on the go!

So sharp, so much fun, and so *on the ball*
How I long to remember, and long to recall:
Endless walks, sun, or snow when I was small...
She'd pick me up when my spirit would fall.

My first real buddy, my first true friend,
Her ears and shoulders she'd always lend;
If I was sad, my pain I'd spend
(But always through her, my heart would mend).

INTERMISSION
But when I was about seven, in 1963,
Something in her changed, so drastically.
She would no longer laugh, (She no longer knew me).

She would wander about, so aimlessly
She would light the gas stove, and let the fire run free!

Her eyes then would gaze, in a wild "combat stare"
She grew mute and confused, (She would "pick" at her hair).

Who was this new stranger, taking over her mind?
Where did her spirit go, what did it find?

From doctor to doctor, this mystery grew,
it was 1965, and still nobody knew
To a state institution eventually,
(Her spirit then faded each day, religiously).

She grew steadily worse, it took six more long years,

I would visit her with my mother,
(We would shed many tears).

Day passes were draining, the public would stare
We'd assist her in the bathroom,
(Comb the knots from her hair).

I wonder how she felt, personality "withered"
Did she realize her melt?
(Were her synapses in a blizzard?)

FINALE
On the thirteenth of April 1971
When the hospital called us, 'twas the weight of a ton
She was terminally losing the battle, and had wasted away,
Lost all faculties, (not her choosing)
She died soon after that day.

I reached for her hand at the bedside,
To say *good-bye, friend* on that fateful day.
She mumbled and stared and *connected*
She mumbled as if to say:
"So long for now Susan, for I'm afraid it's time to take my rest,
'Cause Alzheimer's drained my life away,
(But at least you've inherited my zest!")

REFLECTIONS
Twenty years later, I weep for the past
Fond memories of Ann, (she left the *good life* so fast).
Her suffering, although it was an unfair curse,
Was the stimulus for me to become a nurse.

As I seriously reflect on this draining disease
That robs the brain of freedom cells, and independence ease

I AM ANGRY NO DEFINITE CAUSE OR CURE HAS BEEN FOUND.
ALL THE RESEARCH WON'T TOUCH THE PAIN THAT ABOUNDS.

If I had just one wish that would be granted to me,
I'd want to spend a day with Ann, just her and me.

Her cheerful style, giving nature so gold,
Her best feature "zest", her stature so bold...

(...But who's kidding who...she was taken away in her prime-
A true servant of God, Strong will, lost mind...)

Signed,

"One who can still remember"

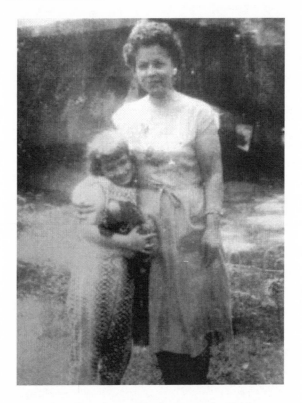

Grandma Ann with Susan, early 1960s

WITH GRATITUDE TO MY MENTORS

Warmest thank yous to all my nursing mentors
Role models I've known and admired
Facilitating choices, paths, risks in my life
Kindred spirits who have kept me inspired.

You've fostered examples, such lessons you've taught
My talent you've nurtured in countless ways
So committed to my ultimate confidence and esteem
No doubt adding zest to my days.

Whether I consulted you
for which career moves I should make
Or if an overdue vacation you'd help me schedule and take
Or your honest *warm fuzzy* every once in a while
And that caring *that a girl* hug and one of a kind smile...

You've been my professors, supervisors, colleagues, and friends
That I could look up to with pride
Respecting your opinions so dear and from the heart
Believing in what ventures I have tried...

So, thank you again from my heart, soul, and mind
Our synergy's priceless, so true,
I'll treasure your honesty, support, and your warmth
But mostly the wisdom of you.

ON SUNSETS

Aren't sunsets amazing?

Just to catch a glimpse of one at prime time
can turn an ominous frown into a smile,
denial into acceptance
anger into friendliness
despair into hope

Yet, to truly appreciate a sunset,
In all its significance, awe, wonder,
(and crisp, deliberate color),
We must
Look inside our core
For just one minute
Remembering why we're here,
Who we are,
What our "purpose" is in life
and then,
As each sunset closes the chapter of the day
Be thankful for all we've got.

I imagine that life with HIV/AIDS is like
Trying to buy high priced,
sold out, fake tickets
For life's last beautiful sunset,
From a swindling scalper
Who, frankly
Doesn't give a damn about you... ·

I imagine that life with HIV/AIDS is like
Life's last loving chapter coming at
the beginning or middle
of a magnificent novel...

I imagine that life with HIV/AIDS is
Premature conversations,
collaborations
and confrontation
with the higher powers...

Life with HIV/AIDS is...
no more
sunset, sunrises,
sun, no more

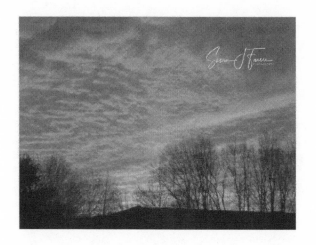

Photo by Susan J. Farese

PLEASE WRITE!

When you have some time,
Please, read the local paper
Observe, if you will...

Any articles
Written for or by nurses?
(I'll bet you there's few)!

They'll quote the doctors
Researchers and drug firms
(Even the public)!

Are we that faceless?
With no credibility?
(I highly doubt it)!

Let's share our brilliance...
and write editorials,
columns, articles!

We are the experts
Who can write about things like
Health care, cholesterol!

We are advocates
The ones who stay with patients
In health or illness

Let's bond together
And write what we know about
We're nursing experts!

MY FRIEND

Your silver bristles
Hang straight, disheveled with oil
(At the nursing home).

Slouched in a wheelchair,
Gazing boldly at nightfall
(What are you thinking)?

They schedule you
To "attend activities"
(No insanity)!

You don't want to sit
With head lowered and frowning
(You've more life to live)!

Let's go for a walk
In the bright sun, you and me
(A new beginning)!

You have the wisdom,
Your experience abounds
(You're my role model)!

Together we'll share
Stories from our lives diverse
(And we shall *connect*)!

More than my patient,
You've grown to become my friend,
(A bond to cherish)!

GRANDPA JOE

Grandpa, a baker died of an asthma attack
In his own kitchen.

A man so gentle,
I remember him vaguely
He died...I was eight.

1964
Now I can remember him,
Kindhearted, at peace.

Hair was gray and thin,
and his hairline receding
(He'd sit on the porch)

He'd pay a nickel
I would spit on my hands,
And style and comb his hair!

His long, roman nose
And his voice, one of a kind
Yes, that's Grandpa Joe!

Schaefer and Budweiser
Camels he smoked many packs!
Ate lots of cashews!

He suffered so much
Allergies to everything
Now, I remember

But it all ended
Asthma and emphysema
Competed with him!

He could hardly breathe
He worked hard all his life,
Never took days off.

Back then there were less
Treatments and procedures to
Make him all better.

(I miss you grandpa,
Even though I was eight then,
I loved you so much!!)

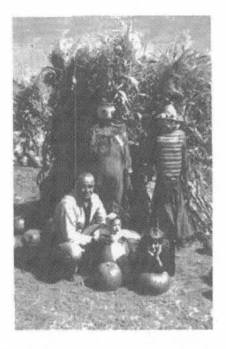

Grandpa Joe, Susan and her brother, 1963

SPOUSAL INTUITION

The ICU twelve hour shift almost through,
At 5:10 PM that day
"Mr. H." was transferred to our *haven*
Confused, impending doom, in disarray.

His charge nurse gave a quickened transfer report
They "couldn't define" what was wrong
He was "just so different" after the Xray,
"he'll be sent via bed now, so long"

Within minutes five, he and bed did arrive,
Then vitals, 02, IV and leads,
His life traveled downhill
Shallow resps, tachy pulse,
Low BP, 02 sat down, indeed.

Sitting upright, so ashen
he said, "I'm not breathing well,
I'm so thirsty nurse, can I have a drink?
PLEASE CALL MY WIFE, AM I GOING TO DIE?"
Then the monitor alarms wailed in sync!

He grew grayer in bigeminy, coughed frothy sputum
and stared,
He trusted this was his last life's sail.
We bolused with Lasix and lidocaine
Did what we could, (to no avail).

Sadly, he coded at 5:25,
Enveloped in V tach and fib rhythms,
Despite ACLS, our team efforts had failed,
Then when everyone left, I stayed with him.

We notified his wife, an invalid, home bound
Her aide brought her in for the viewing,
"He asked for you at the end," I explained
She sighed, hugged me, cried (some renewing).

"But what was so coincidental", her home health aide said,

16

"Was that at 5:15 at home,
Mrs. H. was awakened by a dream while in bed,
She sat up, yelled, "my husband" and moaned".
And so I must tell you to listen actively
To our patients who tell us a story,
Believe in what they're telling us
Believe them, for they know the glory.

Take heed in their words and intuition,
Our mission's to save them above all odds,
But sometimes they've a strong, eerie vision
For the ultimate visit with their gods.

DON'T SHOW, DON'T TELL

Enterprising Creature, lurking deep within,
The chambers and channels beneath one's own skin.

Since its dawn in the eighties
Draining enigma to most
In the prime of their lifetime
Consuming victims as hosts.

So subversive, so sneaky
(Can one detect its sole quest?)
To gnaw at one's persona
To rob one of their zest.

No matter one's skin tone
No matter one's worth-
Affecting worldwide proportions
Upon this our planet Earth.

Risk factors will vary
But share a common thread,
For this unique desperate journey
Spares no one the dread.

Isolation abounds
To those chosen who are stricken
They endure muscle wasting, fatigue (fevers quicken).

Whether presumptive or definitive,
Carrying the virus is grief
It's stigma to all that are seeking relief.

Where will this finish? Where will this end?
How many will perish? Or will science stop the trend?

Unfortunately, these questions can't be answered just yet,
So, treat those who suffer with compassion, not regret.

WE MUST BOND TOGETHER, our prejudice PURGED
UNITED WITH EMPATHY, DEFEATING THIS SCOURGE

INTUITION

Please respect your intuition
And acknowledge every *hunch*
For you will find most certainly,
This "preference" is worth a bunch!

It's that *cozy* yet dangerous *gut, feeling*

That appears every now and then
You cannot explain this phenomenon
You just *know what will happen*...and *when!*

It may be a *look* in a person's eye
(Or a sense of impending doom)
Predicting endless possibilities
...It's the "aura" inside a room.

Whatever this is, be wary and wise,
Don't cast it aside and ignore it...
If you're gifted with intuition, my friend,
Sit back, just relax, and adore it!

SHHHHHH!

I was listening last week in the hospital hall
To what passersby had to say
Unbeknownst to them, I remember their phrases
Wow, this opened my eyes, all the way!

The voices diverse included the Nurse,
Doctor, Pharmacist, Tech, Volunteer,
Patients, their visitors, Phlebotomists alike:
Yes, I heard all the mouthfuls they shared!

You're invited to partake here of some of their words
(Which I gather may seem familiar to you too)
I trust that you soon will join forces with me
(And be wary of your words, tried and true)!

"She's the dysphagia queen of the hospital"
"Are you still on call Saturday night?"

"I am not a type A get me out of this place"
"Hi John, nice tan, those scrubs fit just right!"

"They need a transplant eval on her soon"
"Did they tap him?" "Which room is she in?"
"That guidewire worked like a breeze"
"Did you know she had two dates last week with Edwin?"

"Pick Timmy up later, get something to eat"
"The hemoglobin's up to 16"
"Now it's primary care that we practice"
"I'm exhausted from these treatments, call Jean"

So as you can plainly see, this did a number on me,
And now I'll be more wary and wise
When in the hospital halls you too, I now trust
Shall not chat too much, heed my advice!

20

MATTERS OF HIS HEART

THE BEGINNING
July 19, 1992
4 A.M. phone call Intense, horror, foreboding...
And mom's voice, so shrill...

"We're in the E.R.
Dad's having a heart attack
(When can you fly home)?"

Huge lump in my throat
With quickened pulse I paced and
Somehow, booked the flight...

My thoughts on the plane
Ranged from melancholy to
Fear...to such anger!

How could this happen?
(I just talked to him Tuesday-
Oh, now I recall...)

He stated that day
He "must have been allergic"
to something outside...

He said his throat was
So "warm" like hot tea poured down
to his lungs, he said...

It went away though,
He stopped what he was doing
Went inside to rest...

How we all were fooled This *significant* signal,
Angina, it was

Intermittently
For the next few days or so
Dad wasn't "himself".

Then, after dinner
He went upstairs to sleep
A full day, it was.

1:30 A.M.
Chest pains did wake him
nausea, sweating ...

Doom so impending
He drank some bottled water
-No relief in sight...

He wandered,
looking for insurance I.D. cards
(Get to the E.R.!)

And at the same time
My brother somehow showed up
"Dad, what's the matter?"

"I don't know", dad said,
But something's wrong, I must go
Heart attack, I think"

Dad wanted to drive
He didn't even wake mom,
(No time to waste now!)

My brother drove him
Despite dad's wishes to drive
(What intuition!)

When they both arrived
Dad was ashen and fading-
They triaged at once

Vital signs, O_2
EKGs, labs, consult by
Cardiologist.

Nitroglycerine didn't resolve his pain so

They used TPA...

The "liquid gold" was
used to dissolve the thrombus
Chance for life anew...

Vital signs stable
Transfer to CCU
A new journey ...

FLIGHT HOME
My flight then arrived
I kept wondering if I
would see him alive...

Please, dad, HANG IN THERE!
I won't be able to cope
Without seeing you...

Mom met me at home,
we hugged too briefly and then
Drove off to see him...

CCU VISITS
In the hospital,
I felt I owned the place
I felt in control...

I believe that by being a nurse as well as
his daughter helped us...

I was able to interpret tests and labs and
explain things to them...

I felt sorry for
families without any nurse:
We were fortunate!

My first glance at dad
Proved to be so different
His color still pale

Constantly watching
I reviewed his rhythm strip
when we were chatting.

I placed both of the chairs
So that mom and I could be
As close as we could...

The CCU nurse
explained everything to me,
using nursing terms...

Yes, his enzymes were
extremely high and
His MI ruled in...

He suffered a "jolt"
Anterior-lateral
Yes, he was stable...

In the CCU
primary care prevailed
He'd stay there 4 days...

I felt dad was safe
the care was exceptional
(Was this all a dream?)

STEP DOWN
Dad had no more pain.
They had transferred him to the
Telemetry floor.

He was monitored
to detect any ectopy
By EKG leads...

And during this phase
He was on a heparin drip
To keep him clot free

Dad was such a trip
Ambulating the halls with

His "IV Pole Pet!"

In reality
I was dad's true advocate
And case manager!

I'd make sure that he
would conserve his oxygen
By getting his rest...

If the nurse forgot
Tylenol for his headache
I would remind her...

If he drank something
I would do his I & 0
on a memo pad...

He progressed so well
That the next procedure would
Be cardiac cath!

AFTER MATH, AFTER CATH!
Dad's cath revealed
90% narrowing
in his "L.A.D."

He was stabilized
Then the next plan for him was
Angioplasty.

QUIET
Quiet was when we waited...
waited...
for the results of dad's angioplasty...
waited in a room,
A room with a view

A view for those who prefer
Who prefer to face the *window*
The window rather than the situation...

We waited...

...That was when it was quiet...

AFTER THE ANGIOPLASTY

Dad's procedure was a success.
But the chances
of restenosis
were 25-40%.

That meant, we'd need to wait and see
and cross fingers
and hope
that it was the right thing to do

So, we were optimistic
and he was discharged
and could pursue
life again
on his terms...

and I flew home
(and really started to worry, but kept it to myself...)

AUGUST THROUGH NOVEMBER

From August through November,
I was uneasy...
I knew something *wasn't right*
I couldn't get dad out of my mind...

That intuition would not quit.

However,
Dad was progressing, doing his daily exercising,
losing weight steadily
being *compliant* with medication therapies...
Mom felt great too...
Cooking fat-free foods, walking with dad,
a new lifestyle, a new chance...

"I'm fine", he would always say...even to me... the nurse...
I was worried, but kept it to myself...

And so, dad remained status quo... until

Late October... when he went for a walk
And felt pain in his gut
and a burning in his throat ...
ominous sign...

It was certainly
my worst fear...
Restenosis

That dreaded event that may occur
following angioplasty...

In for an urgent stress test
which he flunked massively...

His EKG showed horrendous changes:
Oxygen was robbed from his heart each minute
Another heart attack was very likely...

This news came on the eve of the presidential election
I would need to fly home once more...
When will this end? What next? Will I be able to cope?
Dad, please do well... I am not ready for this...
I am holding on
to good thoughts only
like childhood memories
At the zoo, going fishing, etc. etc. etc...

CATH #2
He was supposed to *have* a cardiac cath
and another angioplasty

But when they did the cath,
which showed massive restenosis and damage,
nearly all blocked again...

Now,
a decision would be made

In all of twelve short hours...
Dad would need coronary bypass surgery

or else would be high risk
like a time bomb
ready to explode
with severe consequences ...

He cried, we cried, we worried all,
but as a family
were prepared to handle anything we needed to...

Dad's faith was so very strong
that he went to surgery
much like he was going to be playing
in a football game
It would be tough, and a team effort
and we prayed and prayed...

We prayed incessantly ...

Dad was indeed braver than anyone I've ever met that day.
We prayed...

WAITING ROOM BLUES
Listening to
the music from my Walkman
helps me to relax a bit;

I feel set free...
The ensemble a calm peace perhaps
allowing myself to let go...

None of us...Dad, nor Mom, nor I are in control any longer
The pilot of dad's vessels now is another...

A higher power
Controls his new destiny, new heart,
his life anew...

Whether he shall be angina free
Whether he will have quality of life
Whether he shall walk, talk, be merry
Whether he shall LIVE…and be dad again...

Good ole "pop"

life of the party
catalyst
getting things going
then going his way...

Never a complainer,
never a sissy
calm in emergencies
macho man pop...

"They'll never use a saw on me" he said in July
After the heart attack
and through the months after...

They just gave an update...
He's connected to the bypass machine.
Now they are fixing his damaged vessels

I am afraid
So afraid
I am finally dealing with mortality for real

We can only wait... so we will...
(And today was Friday the 13th...)

BYPASS
Well, he is off the bypass
Old blockage
replaced by new enriched blood flow

Like a freeway with a bottleneck
needing relief
and room
for the vehicle
the blood
to pass through
without the narrowing, the stenosis, the killer...

And so, being the educator I am
and caring so for mom
I drew a crude diagram
for her

29

so I could show her
how dad would look
following surgery
the ventilator, EKG leads
chest tubes, IV's
Foley, swan,
pacing wires, dressing

and on and on...
just to take the edge off
and prepare her for the event
of seeing dad
like that...

But mostly to take away my fears

CARDIOTHORACIC SURGICAL INTENSIVE CARE
THE FIRST VISIT (5 PM)
They allowed me to see him
an hour after arriving
in the unit...

I went in first
bracing myself for the worst
prepared to lose it all...
prepared to be afraid...

But his nurse
was the key to my coping

She smiled warmly,
and said
"You're his daughter, the nurse?"

I immediately felt calm and serene
and trusting
and let go
and relaxed and rejoiced and thanked God
and thanked nursing

because her smile
made all the difference...

Dad although a bit pale
had his tubes positioned exactly where
I drew them in mom's picture

He was stable. His lids were closed.
His ventilator breathed for him to ease him back
He slept peacefully

With the nurse at his side who made all the difference ...

2ND VISIT
His nurse, smiling
met me at the door
He was waking up!

Go see him!
softly she said...

Eyelids open, tears falling a bit
ET tube in place
pulse, BP, wedge, stable

I kissed him lightly
and said he did so well,
he did so well indeed

It was over

Just rest, dad, sleep, we love you
Everything went well, dad, get some rest... I'll be back...

THE NEXT DAY

ET tube out
speaking again
a little out of breath
a little in pain...
but otherwise

No one would ever know what he went through
Yesterday

how brave he was...

still pale, from blood loss
blood infusing

potassium infusing
check the monitor

Stop that, you are not the nurse... you are the daughter
relax Susan, relax, be thankful
He's alive
and will be dad again...

CHRISTMAS '92
Six weeks later
Dad and mom boarded a plane
and came to see us this time

No more angina
No more fright
a new man, with a new mended heart

walking each day
healing and feeling stronger

And what a perfect gift
he gave to mom and me

To say thanks

Each of us received
a beautiful, symbolic
gold heart shaped necklace,
hers aquamarine to match her eyes
mine, amethyst...

I call it my purple heart

(He's the one who deserves a medal such as this...)

I'll treasure it always

For it represents
Matters of his heart...Matters of his heart.

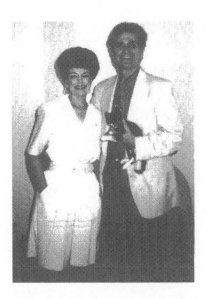

Note from Susan: My parents are now in their mid 80's!

DONNA

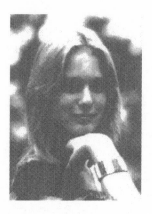

A personal poem to a friend and her family,
after the unfortunate death of her sister from malignant melanoma

She was thirty years old, sadly taken away
In the prime of her life, August 1st was the day.

Why has it happened?
Why was it her turn?
Why the suffering unending?
(From the culprit: "sunburn").

It's not fair that we've lost her, she had much more life to live

(But perhaps, yes up in Heaven –
her glow and presence she'll give.)

She fought hard and hung on, till the very last night.
Her family was with her, when she closed her life's light.

Just one more thought, and then I shall end

Donna's very much *alive*, and she'll continue to send...
Her *connections* to you, inside joy you will feel
From the days she was here, with her energy, her zeal...

So long for now Donna, you'll not be forgotten soon.

We'll miss you and love you...'Til the sun meets the moon...

A letter and eulogy from Susan Lisovicz, (Donna's sister) to the author.

July 1993

Dear Susan,

Donna died when she was just 30. Her battle with cancer typified the way she led her life: even as she was dying, she worried about others. There was little else she spoke of in her final weeks other than the impending birth of my brother Jim's child. (His first baby died after two days.)

She fought her disease with such resistance that we had to keep increasing the morphine so that she could get some rest. But she was stoic about the likelihood of the final verdict. Sloan Kettering was so impressed with her outlook that she was asked to provide counseling to others in the final stage of her illness.

Donna survived her first bout with cancer in 1983. She had passed the critical five-year mark to be considered a "survivor" but discovered a new lump in the winter of 1990. She died August 1, 1991.

We were touched by the outpouring of love in Donna's passing--and the diversity. Flowers, donations, mass cards, food, thoughtful letters, companionship were of great comfort. Your poem was especially touching because of the time, care and sensitivity involved. It means a lot.

A EULOGY

As many of you know, when Donna realized her disease was terminal, she set two goals for herself. One was to live to see the christening of her godson, Phillip. The second was to meet the newest member of the family ... Edward ... born just twelve days ago.

She did both - because she willed herself to do so.

Donna was very weak for Phillip's christening ... so weak that the christening was held at her home. But she still very much wanted to be a part of the occasion. My mother brought her a pretty white dress ... my sister-in-law Laurie did her hair and I did her makeup ... like I did at all her big events. Donna was stoic and peaceful for the ceremony ... and those of us who were there, know we will never witness a christening as meaningful.

Within weeks, as her disease progressed and she slipped in and out of consciousness, there was little else she talked about other than the impending birth of her brother Jimmy's child. She was worried because his first baby had died shortly after birth.

Both events are telling about why this young woman touched so many lives: She was extraordinarily compassionate and extraordinarily brave.

I used to say that Donna always took in strays: cats that were abandoned in the neighborhood and people down on their luck who needed a friend.

That compassion became even more pronounced during Donna's illness. She would often comfort her roommates in the hospital ... women invariably older than herself. She would ring the nurse to make sure the medication was on its way and coax them to think positively. But why was she confined to a hospital bed ... unable to enjoy life like other women her age? Why her? Those were questions I never heard from my sister. What she challenged was the verdict.

Donna wanted to live.

Donna wanted to return to work after a year of debilitating treatment when she didn't have to ... when most people wouldn't dream of it.

Within days, she collapsed.

Donna's struggle against such odds was inspiring. and so was the deluge of love and support that inspired her to keep fighting: her co-workers who left Donna's desk untouched for months in hope that she would return ... the little girls down the street who drew her get well pictures ... my father's carrot juice concoction because beta-carotene helps fight cancer ...
her husband John's unwavering devotion.

She called him her beat ... her heart beat.

Donna had a joy for life and a gentleness that belied her strength. But her essence is best captured in an essay she herself wrote after her first bout with cancer at age 22. I found the essay in a pile of school papers while rummaging through a desk in my parents' house. It was dated September 27, 1984.

There comes a time in everyone's life when they have to face up to certain things about themselves. For some, it may be a fairly young age, while yet for others it could be much later. For me, I started to realize a lot about myself when it was discovered I had cancer.

I guess I've always been a romantic at heart. Ever since I can remember, I always pictured myself married and raising babies with lots of animals running all over the house. When I realized I might never be able to raise any children of my own, it was very depressing for me. I had always thought the miracle of birth was wonderful, and not being able to live it really upset me.

And then there was the fact that I was only 22 years old, and a pretty good chance that I wouldn't be around for my twenty-third. It was then that I realized how much I had taken my life for granted. I loved my life, and I didn't want to face the fact that I had some incurable disease that could take it away from me.

There were so many things I wanted to do. I had never gone horseback riding, water skiing or camping. All of these things came to my mind, and I realized there was so much that I wanted to do.

The support that I received from my family and friends was immeasurable. They had all helped me through the hardest time of my life. After my boss found out what had happened, he immediately phoned my mother with the name of an excellent doctor who practiced in Sloan Kettering Memorial Hospital.

My doctor and all the other doctors who worked with him were exceptional. The time they spent talking to me and examining me was reassuring. I was not nervous the day I was operated on because I had total faith in my doctors.

The operation turned out to be successful ... the cancer had not spread in my body. I would have to be carefully watched for the rest of my life, but that was the least of my worries. I had my whole life to live, and I realized that was all that mattered.

AYAWNA

Her name, Ayawna, Poised, so humble, sensitive
Twelve years "young" she is...

Ebony, smooth skin, so polite to all she meets,
(A poet too...no less!)

So intelligent!
Intuitive, she "connects" With whom she's crossed paths

I'll never forget
Our first meeting, her and I We bonded and smiled...

But this graceful girl Couldn't run or play too much
(She was getting weak)

Her heart and lungs were Deteriorating and
"Wished" for a transplant...

She used oxygen
To help restore her breathing
(No school days... too ill)

Until last week when A wonderful miracle...
"The gift of new life"

Now Ayawna can
Enjoy life's pleasures, once more with us all, again.

Please rest, Ayawna,
And regain your strength so that We can meet again...

July 18, 1992
A Year Ago, Today
By Ayawna Reid

A year ago, today,
I was off and, on my way, In a jet airplane.
My destination: Pittsburgh.
My reason for going: A heart and double lung transplant.
That transplant changed my life,
In a great way,
Exactly just one year ago today.
Before my transplant, there wasn't much I could do. But now I can do much,
Just as much as you.
I play the alto saxophone, and walk a mile a day,
And walk up and down the stairs when I go to school.
I ride my tandem bicycle with friends,
Up and down the street,
And race my cousins on (what seems like) my brand-new feet.
So, you see, I can do much more now,
Than I could just one year ago, TODAY!

My name is Ayawna Reid and I am 12 years old. I would like to thank Susan Farese for letting me contribute a poem to her collection of poems. I would also like to thank all of the people who helped raise money and donated money for my much needed transplant.

NOTE from Susan: Sadly Ayawna passed away in 2005. R.I.P. Ayawna.

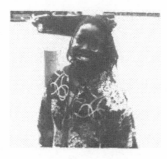

Courtesy photo 1993 Ayana Reid and Family

ODE TO THE WOMAN OF THE '90S

The woman of the '90s, seeks challenges *galore,*
Says "no" with finesse, (even confidence),
when she can't take *any more!*
She deals well with conflict, looks forward to change anew,
Sets goals so she can self-actualize and exists as a role model too!

She manages time (so it won't manage her),
A true leader, inspiring her team,
Communicating with assertion, exuding positive self-esteem!

Besides dressing for success, having insight is her quest
This woman of the '90s is no *coward,*
And with gifts like intuition, zest, smarts, and a heart
She loves life, and she's incredibly *empowered!*

Whether she's your wife, mother or sister or friend
Or aunt, grandma, daughter, or mate
Three cheers for the woman of the '90s
Innovative, so clever...SO *GREAT*

THAT SHINING STAR

I want to be that shining star...
That "breaks through" the glass ceiling and prospers.
Not only with capital ventures ...or marketing skills...
or business wizardry...or savvy.

But with all of those other ingredients.
You know, the "personal triumphs"...
Like real self-esteem,
Self-worth,
Pride,
True confidence,
Spirit, zest, and love...

Letting my "inner child" through the barriers
From time to time

Truly being giving and honest with others (and myself).
Examining, clarifying, and perhaps changing my values
and work ethic.

I want to be that shining star...

(Which route do I take?)

Assertive? Aggressive? Passive-Aggressive?
Selfless? Self-righteous?
(The who's, what's, when's, where's, how's and why's
of the real me...)

It's tough sometimes as each decade passes.
There are new themes, conquests, and identities,
That court, compel and repel us...

Yes, we are into the nineties!

Yes, the nineties are upon us!

Let's combine our powerful forces, seize the moment,
hitch that star!
(It's there, can you see it? Giving us the *You're really* OK blink!

Join me, let's be *us* and forget about "competition"

That lethal, toxic, lonely entity,
Like the sky
When it's dark
Without stars
Like "us"
To shine bright and share light.

I dare us to be... those shining stars...

ODE TO EMILY

Eighty years young and undoubtedly so full of energy
Positive thinking's the name of the game for Grandma Emily
Her smiles are sure to brighten up the gloomiest of days
So proud she is of all of us, our latest snapshots she displays!

Fond she is of baseball, knows the latest scores and stats
She has a flair for fashion
and coordinates outfits in no time flat!
She's up to date on current events, watching late night TV news
She's sure of herself, mighty confident and clearly expresses her views!

What makes her ever so special is her healthy state of mind
Always active, on the go, and to others she's very kind...
Three cheers for gram, an example for all of us to emulate
Please don't ever change, stay the way you are
(Cause to me you're simply great!)

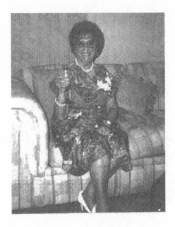

Note from Susan: Grandma Emily passed away in 1998. R.I.P. Grandma

BRENDA: HEROINE AS WELL

(Written after meeting Mrs. Brenda H. Schwarzkopf at a Sigma Theta Tau
convention reception in Tampa, Florida, 14 November 1991)

While your warrior was in Saudi, *being all that he could be*
You endured sandstorms of distance, coped well with dignity...

The nation watched with wonder, awe,
then amazement of his heroics.
(While he planned, led, and executed
those powerful historical moments)

Let us not forget *your* strength
As ambassador for the nation's families
Left behind while Desert Shield and Storm
grew from *concept* to *finality*.

Unending support and courage
During uncertain times was displayed
And validates that spouses or loved ones
Were in fact guardian angels portrayed.

After all is said and done
And when the fanfare eventually ends
Please remember you're truly admired
As a role model by compassionate friends...

NON-DOMINANT DOMINANCE

Don't worry patient...

I will take care of you,

I won't abandon you,

I cherish our bond...

Don't worry patient

...You can weep with ease

...You can say you're scared

In the darkness surrounding.

I am your nurse...

Here to assist you...

To cope with your loss

The loss of your health.

Let's join our forces

To reach our horizons

Protecting our beings

Together we're one...

Note: Written with my non-dominant hand after attending the "Nurturing the Inner Nurse" workshop, given by Dr. Carolyn Chambers Clark.

ABBREVIATION LANE

In health care, nurses all rely upon abbreviations
Shortened words and phrases that deserve consideration
And so to "illustrate" just how they offer information,
I've jotted down a few just for your own notification!

"Ad lib" can stand for "as desired", "before meals" is "A.C."
"BID" means twice a day, "Blood Pressure"? that's "B.P."!

C with a line on top of it means "with", like, "are you "C" me?"
(And we all know "complete blood count" is known as CBC!)
"CHF", "COPD" are problems that require
A "CXR" or chest x-ray to pinpoint where lungs tire!

"Dx" is diagnosis, "D5W" an "IV"
And dyspnea on exertion, simply put is "D.O.E."

The E.M.S. is who you call in an emergency
They'll take you to the "E.R." (be prepared to pay a fee!)

If you're hypoglycemic and you're looking for a test
Fasting Blood Sugars are ordered (also called the "F.B.S.")
Fever of unknown origin's otherwise an "F.U.O."
"F/U is follow-up, "Fe" is short for iron, you know?

"GTT" is drop, were you aware of that or not?
We use "gr" for grain especially if we measure a lot
Another way to say gastronintestinal's "GI"
"GYN's" a shortcut for gynecology, oh my!

Head, eyes, ears and nose and throat is "HEENT"
Did you know that hemoglobin's known as "HGB"?

And if you want to say it's bedtime, "H.S." is the way
"I & O's" intake and output, 24 hours a day

There's a surgical drain, the Jackson Pratt,
it's known as a "J.P." KCL's potassium chloride,
and kilogram's, "KG"

A liver function test is also known as LFT
and LVH is left ventricular hypertrophy!

Ml stands for milliliter, A milligram? that's "mg"
And for all of you math wizards microgram is abbreviated "ug"

Sodium plus chloride yields us salt, NaCl
"NG's" a nasogastric tube (no doubt, we've inserted them well!)
Nothing by mouth is "NPO" and "NOC" is known as night
"O.D." means right eye
and what's more "O.S." means left, not right!

Partial pressure of oxygen abbreviated is P02
Phenylketonuria? We call it P.K.U.!

"QOD" means every other day we do whatever
QI, QA, and TQM yields quality now and forever!

Range of motion exercise? Oh yes that's "R.O.M."
R/O is used to say Rule out by all of us now and then

"S" with a line on top of it clearly means without
And when there's an immediate need for care
"stat" is what we shout
We use the letters "T.I.D." to say three times a day
The Visiting Nurse Association's known as "VNA"

WBC is white blood count and as you can plainly see
I'm so darn tired of writing this "stuff", I'll skip letters XYZ!

This review's complete so now you all can sit back and relax
Abbreviation Lane's the place to curb words to the max!
Enjoy them all and use them freely to your hearts content
And when you do the time you'll save
is more than what you have spent!

S.O.A.P.I.E. FOR ME?

(OR FOR YOU TOO)?

"Soap charting" was in vogue a few years ago
I attended the classes (we all had to go!)

The object was clear and concise information
To cover our "....." in nursing documentation!

"Subjective" was what she or he plainly stated
"I'm cold", "I'm in pain", "Are my lungs not inflated?"
"My chest really hurts, it's a 5 out of 10",
"I can't move my fingers",
"My head aches again!"

Moving on to "objective", it's what you or I see
Either temps, pulses, resps,
(Don't forget the B.P.!)

It's the intake and output, weight kilograms or pounds
But whatever you write be sure it's within bounds!

Next, our nursing "assessments" (our gut feelings) on paper
Another name nursing diagnosis (The ultimate logical caper!)
Potential or actual this or that,
Astute nursing judgments, describing where we're at.

Identification and the verbiage to mix
What we name is the "problem" we're attempting to fix!

Then the "plan" of the day
Is to list what we'll do
And hope the patient's compliant
And we work together too!

"Implementing" nursing orders
Are the key in the game plan of care
Delegated sometimes, carried out with a flair.

And where would we be without "evaluation"?
(Did we effectively institute care for the patient?)

The morale of the story
The key to success
Is to use this logical process
To prevent your duress.

Good luck with this method, upon it you can depend
It works, it's inexpensive
In litigation it will help one defend!

ACLS MEGACODE TESTING: JULY 1991

ODE TO THE TEAM LEADER!

It's Megacode testing time
And you'll be team leading,
Global "boss, honcho, bigwig"
Here's some tips for your heeding!

No matter what the circumstance,
Establish unresponsiveness
Beginning with "ABC's"
Continually assess if you please!

If you study all the algorithms
that prescribe what you're to do,
You'll no doubt be a more self-assured,
confident, team leader, yes you!

Ventricular arrhythmias are lethal yet are tame
When prompt defibrillation precedes the clinician's game

Three times you "zap", then check rhythm and pulse
(Is he still in V-Fib on the screen?)
CPR, IV, EPI, Intubate then,
As you're coding the human machine.

Don't ever forget to assess the airway
When in doubt check it out with the proctor
Breath sounds equal? Bilateral? regular too?
Finesse, whether Nurse, EMT, or Doctor!

Just remember the clues like "chemical the mechanical"
Give a drug, circulate then defib
Whether lido, Bretylium, it's all still the same
To promote avoidance of more V-fib!

Just a few more things,
Remember to start your "drips"
Before you transfer the patient

(Then no irregular heart skips!) ·

Check blood pressure and oxygenation
Then collapse, cause you'll be hero of the Megacode station!

If unsure take "your" pulse Step back, just relax
Team leading's a breeze if you study to the max!

MR. JONES AND THE NURSE PRACTITIONER

Mr. Jones, what you have is hypertension
Borderline, nonetheless, you see,
170 over 100
(Combined lifestyle and heredity?)

I'm afraid your blood vessels are narrowed
So your ticker can't tick its best way
Without compromised optimal output
But I'm so glad you came here today!

Cause with limiting salt and tobacco
And dropping extra pounds there's a way
To limit the load on your ticker
To reduce *after load* come what may!

Here are some measures that can help you
I'll explain them in total, I'm sure,
Feel free to take notes down, and listen
Compliance guarantees nearly a cure.

Diuretics reduce kidney retention
Exercise helps overall
Beta blockers disrupt adrenalin
Vasodilators open blood vessels all.

I hope you're not confused with this wealth of information
Think it over if you'd like during your upcoming vacation
I'm committed to assisting you combat your condition
So you're healthy and wise with longevity
(Through your own volition.)

See you next month, you can update me then
Good luck, keep in touch, fighting hypertension.

UNIVERSAL PRECAUTIONS

Universal precautions mean
That every patient
Must be treated
The same
When it comes to blood and body fluids.

It does not mean
Gloves are not worn
When you draw one's blood!

It does not mean
You can take urine to the lab
Without it being placed
(From your washed and gloved hand)
Into a pouch or bag.
It does not mean
That you can freely Recap needles
Or manipulate them
After they've been in contact with the patient.

Wake up!
All of us in health care.
Let's think prior to acting
In this brave new world
Of universal precautions.

Let's examine our health beliefs
Strongly
Because it is up to us
Health care providers
To don shields
In order to shield
You from me,
Me from you,
Us from them
Or perhaps, them, yes, them, from us.
Universal precautions: think about it, Won't you?
Please?

THE CODE

Bedlam and action
Envelop me in *the code*
...Cardiac Arrest!

Defibrillation
CPR, meds, and treatments
Team leader controls.

We all stand around
The long stretcher amidst us,
It's a sea of hope.

What say you of this?
How do you feel when you're there?
Are you afraid too?

Let's share our feelings
Of this surrealism
Witness to a code.

It's ok to fear
Our own mortality
when life is so fragile

DAY SHIFT

The frenzied pace amidst this place,
Report is nearly starting
I've thirty patients on my team
My mission: meds, treatments, charting!

I'll make assignments, as best as I can, delegating tasks galore
Appropriate within the scope of practice to our team of four...
I'll assess each patient's bio-psycho-social-spiritual needs
Expertly and assertively communicating
with other disciplines indeed!

From room to room on rounds
I'll check the patient's comfort, mood
Are side rails up? Is the environment safe?
Have the trays arrived with warm food?
Are bedside tables near enough so dentures,
glasses, books, they can reach?
Is trash collected from the prior shift?
Any knowledge deficits where I can teach?

And then the IV drips I'll verify
with of course the utmost pleasure
I'm grateful for the "pumps" which
calculate the dose and measure!
Is the solution correct and still on time?
It is marked with initials and date?
A quick look for infiltration, phlebitis,
(it behooves one, before it's too late)!

And lo and behold, as I think I'm caught up,
can you guess what has just occurred?
You were right, two new admissions have arrived
(so for now, my rounds have been deferred)!

It's almost time for lunch now (of course I'll surely miss again)
I'll grab a late tray if I can (and much to my chagrin)!

Who on the team has the narc keys?
I've three patients now in pain...
(And don't forget to call housekeeping
I've done discharge teaching again)!

Someone almost fell in Room 10
but risk management prevailed
Three postop patients just returned from the O.R.
(orders so detailed)!
The call bell rang just now in room 3
(oops I just heard that crash)!
The freshly filled ice water pitcher
pirouetted into the trash!

I'll make the time to read progress notes
and catch up on the plans
And document significant changes
wherever and whenever I should or can!

The time draws near for the end of shift,
(Somehow I feel I left something undone)
But have no fear, there's always tomorrow,
as I welcome the morning sun!

NIGHT SHIFT

Night shift...
So dear to me
Despite
Its circadian disruption

The nocturnal rhythms
sublime,
So inviting, so relaxing...

Making rounds, with flashlight in hand
and night vision intuition,
The serenity envelops me...

Side rails up, call bells within reach
Bedsides tidy
Breathing in sequence...

Snores and noises
(Unspeakable during prime time)
Status quo during night shift...

Gentle and peaceful,
Those who by day
Lurk and cry and pester
And now
Between midnight and 7
Are compliant!

And yearn
For Peace as well...

Alas,
Time to review and verify
and stuff and thin the charts,
Time to read the progress notes!
Finally, a time to put it all together
Like spies looking for the clues of their lives
And if one is truly lucky,

There are some chosen patients
Who decide
It is time,
during night shift,
to ventilate
truly share
opening up the dam
of
their fears, thoughts, feelings...
Even sharing stories
Enhancing our Knowing

Oh, please, I yearn for these nights...
When the nature of nursing
facilitates the connection of lives

MORNING REPORT

Yes, morning report!
Time for new information
About our patients.

Who needs tests today?
Who'll be transferred, discharged?
And who gets to stay?

Name, age, room number
Diagnosis and age too
-More info awaits!

Vitals, I & O
Activity level too
(Don't forget Diet!)

All seem so mundane
They may change but stay the same,
In morning report.

ODE TO THE HOME HEALTH CARE NURSE

Six home visits
I'll make today
And enrich my patients lives as I pass their way...

A trusting relationship with caring I'll build
Autonomy, independence, compassion instilled
I use clinical, management, and teaching skills too
As I organize and facilitate a healthy state for you.

I take a glimpse at your home with a glance
Use all my senses and intuition to enhance
Assessing your needs and matching them with skill
And deliver quality care and emotional support I fulfill.

I connect with your life and bond as well
Meet your significant others, so them too,
I can tell
About this or that treatment, procedure, or meds you'll need,
For biopsychosocial wellness, this I do indeed.

What make me so special, apart from the rest?
I'm a home health care nurse, on my care you can invest
I'm an advocate so ethical, this fact is true
Providing quality nursing care with pride, from me to you!

THE MIRROR IMAGE

Like the bird,
In brisk flight, all over creation,
Dropping in and on creatures
Nurturing and nesting
From one haven to another
At all times, day, or night:

So is...or may be the nurse.

Like the bird,
Who harvests and chirps
(and sometimes wails)
When someone or something invades their turf:

So is...or may be the nurse.

Like the bird,
That flocks with their own kind or others diverse
For flight and frolic
Monitoring all with watchful eye and intuition:
So is...or may be the nurse.

Yet, unlike the bird,
Who's comfortable in the sky and wary of land,
The nurse, uniquely knowing, unafraid,
Commands the "sparrows needing care"
Whether on land, sea, or air
And embellishes these adventures
With flair......unlike the bird
...unlike the bird

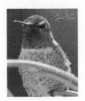

Photo by Susan J. Farese

PATIENT ADVOCATE ...

ASSERTIVENESS CIRCA 1980

I'd like to tell you a story
From my days on the clinical scene,
In the cardiothoracic unit
(When you hear this...don't think I was mean)!

It was something important I had to do
To correct untoward behavior
I'm glad these days as I reminisce
For my *assertiveness* which I now do savor!

Expertly, each evening, to no avail
He'd approach our quaint unit, without any fail.
He'd creep carefully, thought no one would see
And would steal patient's *jello*, tiptoe out, then would flee!

Now I knew the nourishment *fridge*
was for the patients benefit;
(This surgical resident's hunger, didn't seem to want to quit)!
As my ethical *gut feeling* was to nip this bud tonight,
I said farewell to all my fears,
(You'd have laughed if you saw this sight)!

With my watchful eye upon the door
He appeared at his usual time
And alas, inside his ever huge surgical hands
Was a Styrofoam bowl of *lemon-lime*!

And I said, "Doctor so-and-so, I do not care
What you make as a salary,
...or who you know, better yet where you go...
But this buck stops right here now, you see?

The jello's for my patients, only for them, understand?
If you come back and steal again, I'll inform the "jury grand"!
And please, don't think your name will be spared
in night shift report,
You know you were caught *red -handed*

(one more slip and we'll see you in court)!

He grew pale, each second, so anxious and scared
Prepared for the fight or the flight
Said he was sorry, it'll happen no more,
And with that friends, he leaped out of sight!

So the morale of the story
As we all can plainly see
Is to ethically care for our patients
Be an advocate, assertively!

Don't worry about repercussions
Stand up for the principle at hand,
Believe in yourself and your values,
And if need be, take jello in hand!

THE ART OF NURSING:

TO YOUR NOW CLOSED AND HEALING OPEN HEART

Supine, in semi-fowlers ...your heart is now mended
Fingers tremble and point *prn* unknowingly...
What have you been through? What are you thinking?

Your eyes are shut, you are calm, so serene,
(It's over now, for the time being)
The ventilator helps your breathing for now...

Oxygen maintains your pink hue
And a spider web of sorts yields multiple lines and tubes...
From IV's, chest tubes, monitors, leads, foleys
...and pulmonary catheter.

It is oh, so quiet and peaceful, here in the ICU
Yet, at any given moment,
Hell may break loose...
Ah, the awe and wonders of medical and nursing science...

Your midsternal dressing, ruler sized by 4 inches,
has a bit of old drainage underneath...
symbolizing a *simple*, calm, covering of "complex" work
performed by our "team".

Excuse me, I see a few *pvc's* on the monitor.
less than 6 a minute...flip-flop ...just a few...
We'll keep a close watch...

Your belly expands with each heavy
deep mechanical respiration
(A little like a pregnant belly...in...out...in...out)

I see your tattoo on your left arm.
(How amazing...it's a small heart with your initials inside).

Did you know how symbolic that tattoo would be?
Now you have a healing heart with life anew.

Ace wraps adorn both of your legs and thighs
You're another success for us...
All is calm, serene...rest now,
(I'll watch over you) ...

You have an itch, you scratch, I watch
My clinical judgment and the
multiparameter monitors show
that you are stable...
all is well in your world and our world...breathe now, rest now...

We have closed your open heart
You have opened my closed heart...

CAREGIVER

Dedicated to all caregivers of Alzheimer's and memory disorder patients.
Written at Caregiver Day at the Barrington, Largo, Florida.

I, your loving caregiver
Need my own care as well,
So I can be your guiding strength
Hearing stories you may tell...

And follow when you wander
And take the lead at times
Answering your many questions
Listening to your words and rhymes...

I, your loving caregiver
Need time alone for me
To relieve my stress from worry
So your support I can be...

Whether I should write a poem,
Or take a bubble bath
Or go to see a movie
Or walk along some path
Or call a friend and chat a while
Or a big hug receive
Or scream and yell from frustration
(This time I really need)

Please don't misunderstand me
I wear my ribbon with pride
You know you're very special to me
And my love for you I'll not hide.

Just one more thought I ponder
A wish I will convey
Through the trials and tribulations, don't fear ...
I remain your caregiver today...

SORROW SHARED

I am sorry for your loss,
and your pain at this time...

I remember your loved one
(So vividly).
I feel such a powerful presence as I share these words.

Time will pass,
Slowly at first,
Tears will be shed,
And memories will linger.

Losing someone close is a pain so deep,
But the strength and will
To go on
Is much more powerful and pungent.

I cannot wear your shoes,
But would try them on
If you ever need me to.

Call me, when the times are tough,
After time passes yet stays the same.

Because I, too.
Have a loved one I've lost
So long ago,
(But like yesterday)

I remember the pain, the sorrow
The wanting to hold on.

Let's share the sorrow
Together,
Through phone calls, notes or just stopping by
To see each other through.

Because sorrow shared
Can make all. the difference.

TO YOU ALL (RE: 3:45 PM)

TO ALL OF MY PATIENTS:

I'm a nurse
(On "your" side of the health care bridge)
I am afraid,
And I fear
Going to my doctor
At 3:45 PM on Monday.

Only 4 days away...
When he, the doctor,
The presumed medical guru,
Will tell me if I'm OK or not OK
If I must change my lifestyle, habits
And ways of coping with life...

The clock ticks and tocks...
Oh, yes, I am anxious
My pulse quickens
As I read about the possibilities
Of what
I, the nurse
May have wrong with my heart.

TO MY COLLEAGUES:
I have always been intrigued
With studying cardiology.
I've worked on cardiothoracic surgery and telemetry units,
I've taught CPR and ACLS courses.
Even designed a cardiac cath booklet,
And have seen open heart surgery and open heart massage.

...But I must admit,
It may be easier
Being unaware
Of what the possibilities
Could render...

For you see,
My heart is the essence of me
The way I love and live in my world
My caring for my family and friends, clients, and peers
My risk taking; my wisecracking
My poetry, and memories cherished...
Please think of me
On Monday at 3:45 PM.

TO THE DOCTOR(S):
Tick tock, my pulse quickens then calms
I'm in your hands doctor
Show me the difference (Just this once)
Of your nurturing
And caring
The way nurses practice their art and science ...

Don't just tell me it's stress
And give me medication
And have me return for a follow-up visit
So you
Can earn
More money
And satisfy your core, your heart.

TO MY HIGHER POWER:
Please don't allow the doctors
To give me news I cannot handle...
I'm just not in the mood.
Too many life changes lately,
Too many side effects from life's medications
Too many unresolved conflicts
Too much baggage to throw away...in the incinerator
I need time
To make a significant difference
In this, my life

My pulse quickens, my pulse slows
I trust in your judgement
Be easy on me this time; My heart has been broken before
And cannot afford another scar of hurt once more.

Please look in on me
At 3:45 PM Monday.

TO MY HUSBAND:
Think of me On Monday
At 3:45- PM
While you're on your most hectic
Business trip of the year...

I know our bond is strong enough

To carry my fears on a blanket of hope
And let the wind
Take my fears into the gulf
Of Mexico...
You're my support
You love me and I love you.

Our hearts are what melded us together
We are committed deeply to one another
So think of me
And love me even more
On, and despite Monday,
At 3:45 PM.

TO MY FAMILY:
I wish
I could just this once
Be held and rocked
While I weep
Before the news hits me
On Monday at 3:45 PM.

I know my age is young
And that I haven't needed you for awhile
But sometimes
Yes, even full of credentials and nursing experiences
I am very afraid
Of the news to come
On Monday, at 3:45 PM.

A FORMULA FOR SUCCESS

A dash of compassion, a teaspoon of care,
mixed with four bowls of advocate,
stirred four times with dare...

Include change agent seasoning,
professional manner and dress,
All blended with expert clinician finesse!

Then fold in ability, skills, knowledge too.
And sprinkle incredible humor through and through.

Knead batter with patience,
ensure three cups of commitment,
Bake at 350 with savvy with technical equipment.

Refrigerate with loyalty and coat with motivation,
Wrap with ethics, intuition and of course inspiration.

When it's all said and done, there's no profession as diverse
As the art and the science of being a nurse!

Take heed and promote nursing's image with me,
Take pride in how we can be all we can be!

Let's unite one and all, with the formula for success,
It's nursing, it's us, we're a team we're the best!

NURSES UNITE!

Nurses Unite!
Let's show the world in all its entirety
Our uniqueness, our strength

Let's proclaim our vision
And lifetime mission;
To foster health and wellness
on the reality continuum

Let's boast that it is us who can reform health!
With our own
Body of knowledge,
Identity,
Empowerment and self-governance ...

We are not the Handmaidens
Battle-axes
Angels of mercy
or
Playthings
as portrayed on the latest greeting card
or daytime soap opera or evening sitcom...

I dare us to show the world
the unparalleled significant differences
we've made in leaps and bounds...
For years and years

Let's share our compassion, empathy, humor, innovation,
how we love life and support each other

**Nurses, I dare us
to unite!!!**

MY POETRY

I am creative
when I write my poetry...
Less stressed and happy!

With pen in hand
My heart opens up and I
Share all the caring•

Thoughts and images
Memories of yesterday
All fall into place•

One cannot describe
The sheer exhilaration
Of a finished poem...

THE PROCESS

It's the spark...
the ignition...
the moment...
the magic...
the creation...
the passion...
the healing...
the uniqueness...
the sharing...
the humbleness
the solitude...
the brotherhood...
the catharsis...
the insight...
the knowing...
the process...
of
poetry!

SHARING THE CARING

Let's open up our hearts and share the caring
Merge visions, ink and syllables so daring...
Life's fragile, short and sweet,
Grasp rhythm, pace, and beat
Catharsis of emotions we've been wearing.

We've seen it all, the panic, pain, and fears
Of newborns to centenarians in years
From birth to life's demise
Our "knowing" makes us wise
Yet...Prose as *catalyst* releases tears...

Brave and famous poets we need not be
but writing from the heart, that sets us free
Through poems we tell our stories
Share pain, grief, caring, glories
Regardless of our nursing specialty.

No need to build the walls to hide
The memories we've buried deep inside
It's good to let it go, allowing words to flow
Stand back and let the power be your guide.

A TRIBUTE TO NURSING:

IN PRAISE OF NURSES

BY

MOHAN CHILUKURI, MD

Let us sing of Nurses heartfelt and deep,
who labor into the very darkest of nights
fighting the numbness of fatigue and sleep,
drawing strength from reserves unknown - they keep.

These are the true yet oft unsung heroes,
in the long, long halls of healing
curing the weak and sick of curses
of tortured bodies and lost souls,
without whom doctors wander lost,
helpless as bird flightless,
devoid of the uplift of solemn, silent wings.

Behold the Nurse!
The Mother of healing.
The Angel that treads the earth,
The Lady of the lamp,
Whose light shines through tears of sorrow
wiping them with whispers of love and tomorrow,
Whose voice queries the silence of disease,
soothing the inner seething;
Whose gentleness calms the turbulence
of the demented and the diminished,
and whose smile, divine,
brings sparkle and spring to lives
at the dusk of disease and death.

If beauty is devoted action,
there is none more beautiful;

If compassion is divine,
there is none more saintly.
Nursing is much more than a trade or an art.
It is a call from within,
A mission of love to those without,
an inspired act of devotion in one's destiny.
Who is this then who gives of herself
the toil of her sweet sweat;
Who cleanses, calms, medicates, relieves,
injects, assists, smiles, soothes
and touches our very hearts?
She is truly a shining jewel ,
More brilliant than the morning sun,
The very pearl from the oyster of mankind.

A Note:

Dr. Mohan Chilukuri is a family physician who has been in practice since 1985. Dr. Chilukuri has worked closely with nurses since his medical school years and has come to respect them for being able to successfully deal with temporal, physical, and psychological demands that are placed on them in caring for the sick.

Dr. Chilukuri was asked to speak in appreciation of nurses on Nurses' Day in May, 1993. In preparation for that speech, he sat up the night before trying to distill his thoughts and feelings toward nurses. The poem is a result of that process and reflects Dr. Chilukuri's feelings that nurses are an embodiment of compassion, devotion, and endurance.

BONUS SECTION: HAIKU POEMS BY SUSAN

I enjoy writing Haiku and for the past few years have enjoyed teaching my interactive "Capturing Your Creativity With Haiku" workshops to libraries throughout San Diego County.

Haiku is an ancient Japanese form of short poetry comprised of 17 "On" or sounds. The English language version is 17 syllables including 3 lines (5-7-5). Haiku captures a keen single thought or moment and usually has a reference of nature or seasons as well as a juxtaposition or 'aha! moment.

In addition to in-person Haiku workshops, due to the pandemic, I also offer virtual workshops:

https://sjfcommunications.com/upcoming-haiku-workshops/

The following pages contain several Haiku poems inspired by nature and my photography.

I hope you are inspired to write your poems as well!

All the best with your poetry journey!

Susan

MOON AT YELLOW TRAFFIC LIGHT

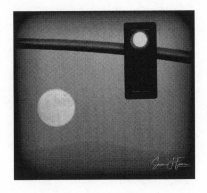

All of a sudden

moon rose, traffic light yellow-

serendipity!

Photo by Susan J. Farese

EGRET AT SANTEE LAKES

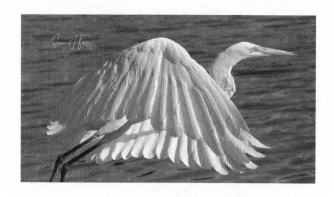

The water glistened

fanned plumage captivating!

Great White Egret soared!

Photo by Susan J. Farese

THOUSAND PALMS OASIS

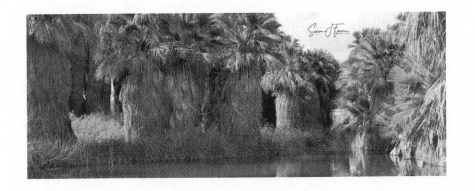

A Spring desert hike

path, date palms, oasis pond

delightful surprise!

Photo by Susan J. Farese

LAKE POWAY OSPREY AND PREY

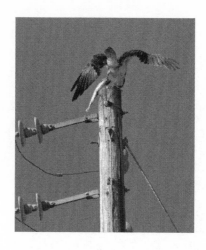

Perched high, above pole

The osprey held on to prey

Then it flew away!

Photo by Susan J. Farese

ODE TO BIRD WATCHING

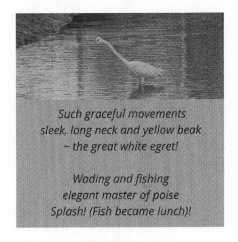

Such graceful movements
sleek, long neck and yellow beak
~ the great white egret!

Wading and fishing
elegant master of poise
Splash! (Fish became lunch)!

Bird Watching is FUN!

Challenging and exciting

(But pay attention)!

All of a sudden

One might grace with their presence

And poof…they fly past!

Camera in hand

Mastering all the settings

Stay still – just don't move!

Nothing like photos

Displaying what you've captured

I LOVE BIRD WATCHING!

Photo by Susan J. Farese

BUTTERFLIES MARVEL

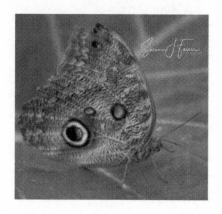

Fickle flutterers

Quick, vividly colorful

Dainty butterflies

They might land on you

If so, they invite your grin

Butterflies marvel!

Photo by Susan J. Farese

HUMMINGBIRDS: MAGNIFICENT CREATURES

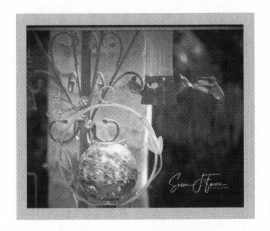

1. Fluttering about

Zooming, oh, so rapidly

Marvelous colors!

2. Hummingbird magic

Unique, beautiful creatures

Don't fly away, stay!

Photo by Susan J. Farese

ABOUT THE AUTHOR

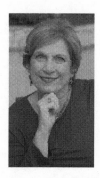

Susan J. Farese, MSN, RN, a native of New Jersey, received her Bachelor of Science (BSN) degree from Widener University and Master of Science (MSN) from Seton Hall University.

Her diversified nursing career includes military and civilian nursing within inpatient outpatient and academic settings- including experience as a clinical nurse in a variety of settings, nurse educator, nurse administrator, legal nurse consultant, and nurse entrepreneur.

Ms. Farese is President/Owner of SJF Communications which provides Public Relations, Publicity, Marketing, Social Media, Websites Speaking, Writing, Filmmaking, Mentoring and Photography.

Susan is a member of Film Consortium San Diego's Advisory Board for San Diego Film Week as well as a member of SAG-AFTRA, American Legion Post 43, Veterans in Media & Entertainment, San Diego Writers Ink and the San Diego Press Club.

Susan gives back to her community as a volunteer mentor at San Diego State University in their Aztec Mentor Program and to her alma mater, Widener University.

Susan's passions include birdwatching, nature photography, writing/poetry, as well as film/tv/theatre. Susan is in awe of hummingbirds, seahorses, heart-shaped items/art and the colors purple and teal.

She lives in sunny San Diego with her husband Mike, daughter Emmy and also is human caregiver to her family's geriatric tuxedo cat Chloe Marie and Betta Fish Alvin Danny Boy.

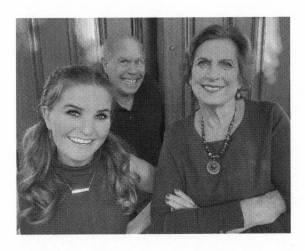

Courtesy Photo – Susan J. Farese

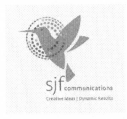

Visit SJF Communications at: https://sjfcommunications.com

Creative Ideas | Dynamic Results

@sjfcommo on Twitter and Instagram

@SJFCommunications on Facebook

Made in the USA
Columbia, SC
08 August 2021